I0095986

GET THE JUICE!

ISBN:978-1-952701-52-8

Published By Impel Publishing

Contents

Introduction

I Got the Juice – And Now, So Will You!

Let's be real—these days, everybody wants the *juice*. You've probably heard the phrase tossed around: "She got the juice," "He got the juice." It means someone's got that *something special*—that glow, that energy, that power. Well guess what? When it comes to health, energy, and real results... **I got the juice**—and I'm here to make sure **you get it too**.

This book isn't just about tossing some fruit in a blender and calling it a day. *I Got the Juice* is your **go-to guide for juicing right**—with intention, flavor, purpose, and power. Inside these pages, you'll learn:

- How to juice properly and get the most out of every ingredient

- What the **color of your juice** says about the nutrients you're getting

- How to **adjust your recipes** based on how your body feels

- Which fruits and veggies give you energy, help with detox, boost your skin, or calm your nerves

- And most of all—how to make juicing fun, easy, and something you actually want to do every day

This isn't just another wellness book full of rules and routines. This is your **juice life manual**—equal parts science, soul, and sass. Whether you're a total beginner or a seasoned green-juice warrior, *I Got the Juice* will inspire you, guide you, and maybe even make you laugh while your cells thank you for the nutrient party you're about to throw.

So grab your glass, power up your juicer, and let's turn that produce pile into pure magic. Because starting now...

You got the juice, too.

Chapter 1: Juicing and the Body's Natural Healing Power

Juicing is more than a health trend—it is a natural therapy that supports the body's ability to heal from the inside out. When fresh fruits and vegetables are juiced, they release a concentrated dose of vitamins, minerals, enzymes, and phytonutrients that are immediately bioavailable, meaning they can be quickly absorbed into the bloodstream. This fast delivery of nutrients plays a vital role in nourishing cells, restoring balance, and triggering the body's own healing processes.

One of the primary ways juicing aids healing is through detoxification. Every day, the body is exposed to environmental toxins, processed foods, and stress. The liver, kidneys, and lymphatic system work hard to remove these harmful substances, but they can become overwhelmed over time. Juicing supports these organs by providing nutrients that assist in cleansing—such as chlorophyll from leafy greens, which purifies the blood, and citrus fruits like lemon, which help flush the liver. When the body is free from toxic overload, it can function more efficiently and begin to repair itself.

Another healing benefit of juicing is reducing inflammation. Chronic inflammation is at the root of many illnesses, including heart disease, arthritis, and autoimmune conditions. Juicing anti-inflammatory foods like turmeric, ginger, cucumber, and celery can help reduce swelling and soothe the body. These ingredients contain compounds that combat free radicals and lower inflammatory markers, helping tissues regenerate and improving joint and organ function.

Juicing also plays a powerful role in immune health. Fruits like oranges, berries, and kiwi are rich in vitamin C, while greens like spinach and kale offer a wide range of immune-supporting micronutrients. The live enzymes present in raw juice help improve digestion and absorption of these nutrients, ensuring that the immune system is well-fueled to fight off infection and speed up recovery.

Moreover, juicing gives the digestive system a rest while still delivering essential nutrition. Because the fiber is removed, the stomach and intestines don't have to work as hard to break down food. This can be especially beneficial for people with chronic gut issues, such as bloating, irritable bowel syndrome, or leaky gut. Giving the digestive system a break allows it to repair damaged tissue while still receiving the nourishment it needs to heal.

From detoxifying the system and reducing inflammation to strengthening the immune system and improving digestion, juicing offers a direct path to better health. When used consistently and wisely, juicing can be a valuable tool in restoring balance, energy, and vitality to the body.

Chapter 2: The Power of Color.

- Green (Spinach, Kale, Cucumber): Detoxifies and provides chlorophyll for cleansing the blood.
- Orange (Carrots, Oranges, Sweet Potatoes): Rich in beta-carotene for vision and immune support.
- Red (Beets, Apples, Watermelon): Boosts circulation and heart health.
- Purple (Purple Cabbage, Blueberries, Grapes): High in antioxidants for anti-aging and brain health.
- Yellow (Pineapple, Lemon, Yellow Peppers): Aids digestion and supports liver function.

Green Fruits and Vegetables

Green fruits and vegetables are among the most powerful foods we can eat for healing, energy, and longevity. Packed with vitamins, minerals, antioxidants, and chlorophyll, these vibrant foods are natural tools for supporting nearly every system in the body—from digestion and detoxification to immunity and cellular repair. Their signature green color is due to chlorophyll, the pigment that allows plants to absorb sunlight and convert it into energy through photosynthesis. In the human body, chlorophyll helps cleanse the blood, improve oxygen transport, and reduce inflammation.

One of the most well-known green vegetables is **spinach**. Rich in iron, vitamin K, magnesium, and folate, spinach supports healthy blood, strong bones, and brain function. Its high antioxidant content helps protect the body from free radical damage. Another powerful leafy green vegetable is **kale**. It is loaded with vitamins A, C, and K, calcium, and fiber. Kale is especially helpful for reducing inflammation and supporting eye and heart health.

Broccoli is another green vegetable known for its ability to support detoxification. It contains a compound called **sulforaphane**, which helps the liver neutralize toxins. It also supports the immune system and is high in fiber for gut health. **Cucumber**, though often overlooked, is incredibly hydrating and contains compounds that help soothe inflammation and flush out toxins from the kidneys.

Among green fruits, **kiwi** stands out for its high vitamin C content, which strengthens the immune system and supports skin repair. Kiwi also contains digestive enzymes that help break down food and improve gut health. **Green apples** provide fiber and pectin, which help regulate blood sugar and keep the digestive system moving. They are also rich in antioxidants that protect cells from damage.

Avocados, although technically a fruit, are full of healthy fats, especially monounsaturated fat, which supports brain and heart health. They are rich in potassium and vitamin E and help reduce inflammation throughout the body. **Green grapes** are another powerful fruit packed with resveratrol and other polyphenols that support healthy circulation and protect the skin and brain from aging.

What gives all of these green foods their color is chlorophyll. In the human body, chlorophyll has been found to help with detoxification, wound healing, and even the reduction of harmful bacteria. It also supports the production of red blood cells, which means more oxygen can be carried throughout the body for energy and cellular repair.

Green fruits and vegetables provide vital nutrients that the body needs to detoxify, protect itself, and function optimally. By regularly including green foods like spinach, broccoli, kiwi, and avocado in your diet, you can experience improved energy, a stronger immune system, and better overall wellness. The vibrant green on your plate is more than just color—it's a signal of life-giving, healing power.

Orange Fruits and Vegetables

Orange fruits and vegetables are more than just bright and beautiful—they are nutritional powerhouses that play a key role in supporting the immune system, protecting vision, reducing inflammation, and even preventing chronic disease. Their rich, vibrant color comes from powerful natural pigments called carotenoids, especially beta-carotene, which the body converts into vitamin A. This essential nutrient is critical for healthy eyes, skin, and immune function.

One of the most well-known orange vegetables is the carrot. Carrots are packed with beta-carotene, which gives them their orange hue. Once in the body, beta-carotene is converted into vitamin A, helping to maintain healthy vision, especially night vision. Carrots also support skin health and help strengthen the immune system. In addition, they contain antioxidants that fight inflammation and protect cells from aging.

Another powerful orange vegetable is the sweet potato. Sweet potatoes are rich in fiber, vitamin C, potassium, and beta-carotene. They help regulate blood sugar levels, support heart health, and provide long-lasting energy. The fiber in sweet potatoes also supports gut health, while their antioxidants protect the body against harmful free radicals.

Pumpkin, another orange vegetable, is not only festive but highly nutritious. It's rich in beta-carotene and low in calories, making it an excellent food for supporting weight management, immunity, and skin health. Pumpkin seeds also provide zinc, which is vital for healing and immune support.

On the fruit side, oranges are the most popular and well-known orange fruit. Oranges are famous for their high vitamin C content, which is crucial for immune defense, skin repair, and collagen production. They also contain flavonoids and antioxidants that support heart health and reduce inflammation.

Mangoes are another delicious orange fruit, loaded with vitamins A and C, as well as digestive enzymes that help break down food. Mangoes are also a great source of fiber, which supports a healthy gut and helps control blood sugar levels.

Papayas are rich in beta-carotene, vitamin C, and an enzyme called papain, which helps with digestion and inflammation. Papayas support healthy skin, boost immunity, and may aid in healing from injuries and illnesses.

What gives all of these orange fruits and vegetables their color is a group of plant compounds known as carotenoids—especially beta-carotene, alpha-carotene, and lutein. These antioxidants not only provide the orange pigment but also protect cells from oxidative damage, slow down aging, and reduce the risk of diseases like cancer and heart disease.

Orange fruits and vegetables are essential for maintaining good health. They support vision, immunity, digestion, and skin health while protecting the body from inflammation and disease. Adding foods like carrots, sweet potatoes, oranges, and mangoes to your daily diet is a delicious and powerful way to help your body thrive. The orange color on your plate is a sign that you're feeding your body the nutrients it needs to heal, protect, and grow strong.

Red Fruits and Vegetables

Red fruits and vegetables are more than just eye-catching additions to your plate—they are packed with powerful nutrients that promote heart health, fight inflammation, and protect the body from chronic illness. Their deep red color comes from natural plant compounds called **anthocyanins** and **lycopene**, both of which have strong antioxidant properties that help the body heal and stay healthy.

One of the most popular red vegetables is the **beet**. Beets are rich in **nitrates**, which help improve blood flow, lower blood pressure, and increase oxygen delivery to the muscles and brain. They also support liver detoxification and contain **betalains**, which give beets their deep red color and are known for their anti-inflammatory and detoxifying effects.

Tomatoes are another red vegetable (technically a fruit) packed with **lycopene**, an antioxidant that supports heart health, reduces the risk of certain cancers, and protects the skin from sun damage. Lycopene becomes even more potent when tomatoes are cooked, making sauces and soups just as beneficial as fresh tomatoes.

Red bell peppers are high in **vitamin C**—even more than oranges—and contain **beta-carotene**, which supports eye and skin health. They also have antioxidants that help reduce inflammation and protect against aging.

On the fruit side, **strawberries** are rich in vitamin C, fiber, and antioxidants. They help protect the heart, support the immune system, and promote healthy skin. **Cherries** are known for their anti-inflammatory properties and can help reduce muscle soreness and support joint health. **Red grapes** contain **resveratrol**, a powerful compound that supports heart health, improves blood circulation, and may slow down aging at the cellular level.

Watermelon, another red fruit, is made mostly of water, making it highly hydrating. It also contains **citrulline**, which supports blood vessel health and improves circulation. Its red flesh is due to lycopene, which has antioxidant properties that protect the heart and skin.

The red color in these fruits and vegetables comes primarily from **anthocyanins** and **lycopene. Anthocyanins**, found in strawberries, red cabbage, and cherries, are antioxidants that help fight oxidative stress, which contributes to aging and disease. **Lycopene**, found in tomatoes and watermelon, has been shown to support prostate health, reduce the risk of heart disease, and protect the skin from damage.

Red fruits and vegetables are essential for a strong and vibrant body. They protect the heart, improve circulation, reduce inflammation, and provide key nutrients that support the immune system and slow the aging process. By including red foods like beets, tomatoes, strawberries, and red peppers in your daily meals, you're giving your body a rich supply of healing compounds that promote long-term health and wellness.

Red Fruits and Vegetables

Purple fruits and vegetables are not just beautiful to look at—they are some of the most nutrient-dense and healing foods on the planet. Their rich, deep color comes from powerful plant compounds called **anthocyanins**, which are natural antioxidants that help fight inflammation, protect cells from damage, and support overall health. Including purple produce in your daily diet can strengthen your heart, brain, and immune system, while also slowing the aging process.

One of the most well-known purple vegetables is **purple cabbage** (also called red cabbage). It's packed with **vitamins C and K**, fiber, and anthocyanins. This combination supports a strong immune system, healthy bones, and a well-functioning digestive tract. The antioxidants in purple cabbage also protect against chronic inflammation, which is linked to many diseases, including arthritis and heart disease.

Eggplant is another powerful purple vegetable. Its deep purple skin contains **nasunin**, an antioxidant that protects brain cells from damage. Eggplants are also rich in fiber and low in calories, making them great for digestion and weight management. Their ability to support heart health and reduce cholesterol levels makes them a smart choice for long-term wellness.

In the fruit category, **blueberries** stand out as a superfood. They are loaded with antioxidants and are well-known for their ability to improve brain function, memory, and focus. Blueberries also support healthy blood sugar levels and improve heart health.

Blackberries and **purple grapes** are other examples of purple fruits rich in anthocyanins and resveratrol—compounds that support healthy aging, improve circulation, and reduce the risk of cardiovascular disease. These fruits also contain fiber and vitamin C, which support the immune system and digestive health.

Plums are sweet purple fruits that support digestion, reduce inflammation, and offer antioxidant protection. Their natural compounds help keep cells healthy and protect the skin from signs of aging.

What gives all of these fruits and vegetables their **purple color** is a group of flavonoids known as **anthocyanins**. These natural pigments not only create the vibrant hue but also protect the plant from environmental damage. When humans eat anthocyanin-rich foods, the same protective benefits are passed on—fighting oxidative stress, strengthening blood vessels, and protecting the brain and heart.

Purple fruits and vegetables are some of the most healing foods available. They protect the brain, strengthen the heart, support digestion, and help the body fight inflammation and disease. By including foods like purple cabbage, eggplant, blueberries, and grapes in your daily diet, you're giving your body powerful antioxidants that help it heal, age slower, and stay strong. The rich purple color on your plate is more than just attractive—it's a sign of deep nourishment and natural protection.

Chapter 3: Juicing for Common Health Goals

- Weight Loss: Low-calorie, nutrient-dense juices help curb cravings.
- Energy Boost: Juices with citrus and greens improve stamina and vitality.
- Detoxification: Ingredients like ginger, lemon, and dandelion root assist in liver cleansing.
- Glowing Skin: Juices with cucumber, aloe vera, and berries hydrate and nourish the skin.

Juicing for Weight Loss: How Low-Calorie, Nutrient-Dense Juices Curb Cravings and Burn Fat

In today's fast-paced world, many people struggle with food cravings, weight gain, and low energy. Often, these issues are tied to poor nutrition, over-processed foods, and a lack of essential vitamins and minerals. One powerful, natural way to address these problems is through juicing. Specifically, **low-calorie, nutrient-dense juices** can be a game-changer for those looking to lose weight and take control of their health. These juices provide the body with a flood of nutrients while keeping calories low—helping to reduce hunger, curb cravings, and boost metabolism. (Dense juices are juices that have a high concentration of solutes, such as sugars or fruit pulp, making them weigh more per unit volume compared to less dense juices. This means a dense juice will have more "stuff" packed into the same space)

When the body lacks key nutrients, it sends signals in the form of cravings—especially for sugar, salty snacks, or heavy carbs. However, these cravings are often a cry for **vitamins, minerals, or hydration**, not junk food. Low-calorie juices made from ingredients like spinach, cucumber, celery, lemon, ginger, and apples deliver an abundance of **micronutrients** that the body is often missing. Once these needs are met, the urge to overeat or snack constantly often fades.

One of the main reasons juicing supports weight loss is that it gives you a high concentration of nutrients without excess calories. For example, a green juice made with cucumber, kale, green apple, and lemon might contain fewer than 100 calories—but it's rich in **vitamin C, iron, potassium, magnesium**, and powerful antioxidants. This makes it easy to nourish the body while staying in a calorie deficit, which is necessary for weight loss.

In addition to reducing cravings, nutrient-dense juices also help regulate **blood sugar levels**. Many people experience energy crashes and intense hunger when their blood sugar spikes and then suddenly drops after eating refined carbs or sugar. Juices made with greens, low-sugar fruits, and fiber-rich vegetables help stabilize energy and prevent these roller-coaster hunger cycles. This makes it easier to avoid overeating and stay on track with a healthy eating plan.

Juicing also supports **detoxification**, which is a key part of healthy weight loss. When the body is burdened with toxins from processed foods, chemicals, and poor digestion, it holds onto fat as a protective buffer. Juices containing ingredients like **lemon, parsley, ginger, and dandelion greens** help cleanse the liver, kidneys, and digestive tract, making it easier for the body to release stored fat and eliminate waste.

Moreover, the hydration that juices provide plays a huge role in appetite control and metabolism. Many people confuse **thirst for hunger**, leading them to eat more when their body actually needs fluids. Fresh juices hydrate the body deeply, which can help reduce false hunger cues and keep metabolism running efficiently.

Low-calorie, nutrient-dense juices are a powerful tool for weight loss and appetite control. They nourish the body at the cellular level, reduce unhealthy cravings, balance blood sugar, support detoxification, and keep you hydrated—all without adding excess calories. When used consistently as part of a balanced lifestyle, juicing can help you feel full, energized, and on the path to sustainable weight loss and vibrant health.

Juicing for Energy: How Citrus and Greens Boost Stamina and Vitality

Fatigue and burnout are becoming more common, many people are searching for natural ways to regain their energy, focus, and vitality. One of the simplest and most effective solutions lies in the power of **fresh juice made from citrus fruits and leafy greens**. This vibrant combination floods the body with bioavailable nutrients, oxygen-rich compounds, and natural enzymes that promote sustained energy, reduce fatigue, and enhance physical and mental performance.

Unlike energy drinks or caffeine, which provide a temporary boost followed by a crash, **juicing provides real, cellular-level nourishment** that supports the body's natural energy systems. Citrus fruits like **oranges, lemons, limes, and grapefruits** are rich in **vitamin C**, a nutrient essential for adrenal health and immune function. The adrenal glands, which produce energy-regulating hormones, rely on vitamin C to function properly. When you fuel your body with fresh citrus juice, you're giving your adrenal system a powerful boost—helping to fight fatigue and increase stamina.

Citrus fruits also contain **natural sugars** that are easily absorbed by the body, providing a quick source of clean energy without the crash that comes from refined sugars. In addition, they're loaded with **electrolytes like potassium and magnesium**, which help maintain proper hydration and nerve function—key factors in physical endurance and mental clarity.

Greens like **kale, spinach, parsley, celery, and wheatgrass** are rich in **chlorophyll**, the green pigment that allows plants to convert sunlight into energy. When consumed, chlorophyll helps increase the number and quality of red blood cells, which improves the body's ability to carry oxygen. More oxygen to your muscles and brain means **greater energy, better endurance, and faster recovery** after activity.

Green vegetables are also packed with **B vitamins, iron, and magnesium**—all nutrients vital for converting food into usable energy at the cellular level. B vitamins help support metabolic function, while iron is necessary for preventing fatigue caused by low red blood cell count. Magnesium helps regulate muscle function and supports relaxation, which is important for restoring energy after physical or mental stress.

When citrus and greens are juiced together, the result is a refreshing, alkalizing drink that wakes up the body, refreshes the mind, and provides a sustained sense of vitality. For example, a juice made from **spinach, parsley, cucumber, lemon, and green apple** can offer a powerful energy boost without the jittery side effects of caffeine. Or a juice with **kale, grapefruit, ginger, and celery** can stimulate circulation, reduce inflammation, and give the body a clean, focused sense of stamina.

Juicing with citrus and greens is a natural and effective way to enhance energy, build stamina, and restore vitality. These ingredients nourish the cells, support oxygen flow, balance hormones, and provide clean fuel for both the body and mind. Whether you're feeling sluggish, overworked, or simply looking for a more vibrant lifestyle, adding citrus and green juices to your daily routine can provide a lasting source of energy and wellness from the inside out.

Juicing for Detox: How Ginger, Lemon, and Dandelion Root Cleanse the Liver and Renew the Body

The liver is the body's main detoxification powerhouse. It filters the blood, breaks down toxins, processes nutrients, and helps eliminate waste from the body. In today's world, with the constant intake of processed foods, environmental chemicals, medications, and stress, the liver can become overburdened. This is where **juicing with powerful natural ingredients like ginger, lemon, and dandelion root** comes in. These ingredients have been used for centuries to support liver health and are now widely recognized for their role in **cleansing the liver and aiding overall detoxification.**

Lemon: Alkalizing and Detoxifying

Lemon is a citrus fruit known for its cleansing and alkalizing properties. Despite its acidic taste, lemon has an **alkaline effect on the body** once metabolized, which helps balance the body's pH levels. Its high content of **vitamin C** and **citrus bioflavonoids** helps stimulate the liver's natural enzymes and promote bile production. Bile is essential for breaking down fats and carrying toxins out of the body through the digestive tract.

When juiced, lemon helps **flush out waste**, cleanse the blood, and support digestion—three major pathways of detoxification. Starting the day with warm lemon water or a juice blend that includes lemon can wake up the liver and jumpstart the body's detox functions.

Ginger: Anti-inflammatory and Digestive Support

Ginger is a spicy root known for its powerful **anti-inflammatory and antioxidant properties**. It aids detoxification primarily by supporting digestion and circulation—two vital processes that work closely with the liver. A healthy digestive system ensures that toxins are efficiently eliminated from the body, while good circulation ensures that the liver receives fresh, oxygen-rich blood.

Ginger also contains **gingerol**, a compound that stimulates digestion and promotes the production of enzymes that help the liver break down toxins. Additionally, ginger reduces bloating and gas, making detox juice blends more comfortable to digest, especially for those with sensitive stomachs. When juiced with lemon and greens, ginger adds warmth and enhances the body's ability to release stored toxins.

Dandelion Root: A Traditional Liver Tonic

Dandelion root may not be as popular in the kitchen as lemon or ginger, but it is one of the most effective natural **liver tonics**. Used in herbal medicine for centuries, dandelion root stimulates bile production, supports liver cell regeneration, and helps the body eliminate waste through the kidneys and colon.

It is rich in **inulin**, a type of prebiotic fiber that feeds healthy gut bacteria and promotes digestion—both essential for the detoxification process. Dandelion root also acts as a **diuretic**, helping to flush out excess water and toxins from the bloodstream. When juiced or made into a tea and added to detox blends, dandelion root can provide a powerful boost to liver function and full-body cleansing.

The Synergy in Juicing

When combined in a juice, **ginger, lemon, and dandelion root work synergistically** to cleanse the liver, stimulate digestion, reduce inflammation, and promote toxin elimination. These ingredients not only support the liver directly, but they also help clear the lymphatic system, improve circulation, and provide antioxidants that protect cells from damage during the detox process.

A juice blend of **lemon, ginger, dandelion root tea, cucumber, and green apple** can be a powerful daily detox drink. It's refreshing, healing, and gives the body what it needs to renew itself naturally and gently.

Juicing with ingredients like **ginger, lemon, and dandelion root** is one of the most effective ways to support the liver and assist the body's natural detoxification systems. These potent plants help cleanse the blood, stimulate digestion, and encourage the removal of built-up waste. By incorporating them into your juicing routine, you're not just drinking a healthy beverage—you're giving your liver the tools it needs to restore balance, energy, and long-term wellness from within.

Juicing for Radiant Skin: How Cucumber, Aloe Vera, and Berries Hydrate, Heal, and Nourish from Within

Glowing, healthy skin is not just a result of good genetics or the right skincare products—it's a reflection of what's happening inside the body. Proper hydration, nutrient intake, and detoxification all play a critical role in the health and appearance of your skin. One of the most natural and effective ways to support skin health from the inside out is through **juicing**. Juicing with ingredients like **cucumber, aloe vera, and berries** delivers hydration, antioxidants, and essential nutrients directly to your cells, helping you achieve a more radiant and youthful complexion.

Cucumber: Nature's Hydration Hero

Cucumber is over **95% water**, making it one of the most hydrating vegetables you can consume. Hydration is key for supple, elastic, and glowing skin. Without enough fluids, the skin becomes dull, dry, and more prone to fine lines. In addition to water content, cucumbers contain **silica**, a trace mineral that supports collagen production and strengthens connective tissue, helping skin stay firm and smooth.

Cucumbers also offer **anti-inflammatory properties** that can help calm puffiness and reduce redness, especially beneficial for people with sensitive or irritated skin. When juiced, cucumber acts as a cooling, hydrating base that refreshes the body and replenishes skin cells.

Aloe Vera: Soothing and Rejuvenating from the Inside

Aloe vera is widely known for its topical skin benefits, but it also works wonders when consumed internally. Aloe juice contains **vitamins A, C, and E**, all of which are essential for healthy skin repair, elasticity, and protection from damage caused by sun and pollution. It also contains **plant sterols** and **amino acids** that help reduce inflammation and promote healing.

Drinking aloe vera helps moisturize the skin from within, reduce acne and irritation, and speed up the skin's natural repair process. It also aids in digestion and detoxification—two essential processes for clear, glowing skin. A sluggish digestive system can lead to toxin buildup, which often shows up as breakouts, dullness, or irritation. Aloe helps cleanse the gut, improving nutrient absorption and clearing the path for healthier skin.

Berries: Powerful Antioxidants

Berries like **blueberries, strawberries, and blackberries** are packed with **antioxidants**, particularly **vitamin C**, which is vital for the production of

collagen, the protein responsible for firm, youthful skin. Berries also contain **anthocyanins**, pigments that fight free radicals and oxidative stress, both of which contribute to premature aging, wrinkles, and uneven skin tone.

Regularly juicing with berries helps protect the skin from UV damage, improves circulation, and enhances the skin's natural glow. Their high fiber content (especially when blended, rather than strained) also supports gut health, which is closely linked to skin health through the gut-skin connection.

The Glow-Up Combo

Juicing cucumber, aloe vera, and berries together creates a powerful skin-nourishing elixir. This trio delivers hydration, soothes inflammation, floods the body with antioxidants, and supports digestion—all crucial components for clear, radiant skin. A simple recipe could include:

- 1 cucumber

- ½ cup aloe vera juice or fresh aloe gel

- ½ cup blueberries or strawberries

- Juice of ½ lemon (optional for added vitamin C)
  Blend or juice these ingredients and enjoy daily for best results.

Glowing skin starts from within, and **juicing with cucumber, aloe vera, and berries** is a simple, effective way to nourish your skin with the hydration, nutrients, and antioxidants it needs to thrive. These ingredients support collagen production, reduce inflammation, flush out toxins, and promote a clear, radiant complexion. By making skin-focused juices a regular part of your routine, you're not only improving your outer appearance—you're investing in whole-body wellness and vitality.

Chapter 4: Getting Started with Juicing

Start simple. You don't need fancy equipment or hard-to-find ingredients. Choose 3-5 vegetables and 1-2 fruits for sweetness. Here are some beginner-friendly combo examples below:

- Carrot + Apple + Ginger
- Cucumber + Pineapple + Mint
- Beet + Orange + Lemon

Even though there are so many different veggies and fruits out there it can be helpful to have a guide of veggies and fruits that are great for juicing, especially if you have never juiced before. Here is a list of Vegetables and Fruits to get you started.

Top Vegetables for Juicing

Vegetables for Juicing & Their Health Benefits

1. **Spinach**
   Benefits: Rich in iron, folate, and chlorophyll. Supports red blood cell production, detoxification, and energy levels.

2. **Kale**
   Benefits: High in vitamins A, C, and K, as well as calcium and antioxidants. Boosts immunity, bone strength, and reduces inflammation.

3. **Cucumber**
   Benefits: Over 95% water. Hydrates the body, flushes out toxins, and soothes the digestive system and skin.

4. **Celery**
   Benefits: A natural diuretic and anti-inflammatory. Supports digestion, reduces bloating, and lowers blood pressure.

5. **Carrots**

     Benefits: High in beta-carotene (vitamin A), which supports eye health, skin, and immune function.

6. **Beets**

     Benefits: Rich in nitrates for improved blood flow, detoxifies the liver, and boosts stamina.

7. **Parsley**

     Benefits: Packed with vitamin C, iron, and chlorophyll. Acts as a natural detoxifier and supports kidney health.

8. **Dandelion Greens**

     Benefits: Powerful liver cleanser and diuretic. Supports digestion and removes toxins through the liver and kidneys.

9. **Zucchini**

     Benefits: Low in calories, high in water and vitamin C. Good for skin, digestion, and hydration.

10. **Fennel**

     Benefits: Aids in digestion, reduces bloating, and has anti-inflammatory properties.

11. **Swiss Chard**

     Benefits: High in magnesium, potassium, and iron. Supports blood sugar balance and bone health.

12. **Broccoli**

     Benefits: Contains sulforaphane, which helps detoxify the liver and supports hormone balance.

13. **Cabbage (especially red or purple)**

     Benefits: Great for gut health, high in fiber and vitamin K. Supports digestion and reduces inflammation.

14. **Romaine Lettuce**
    Benefits: Mild-tasting and hydrating. Contains folate, vitamin C, and potassium for heart and nerve function.

15. **Sweet Potato (small amounts)**
    Benefits: Provides beta-carotene and fiber. Supports vision, skin health, and fullness.

16. **Tomatoes**
    Benefits: Rich in lycopene, an antioxidant that supports heart health and reduces oxidative stress.

17. **Bell Peppers (especially red or yellow)**
    Benefits: High in vitamin C and antioxidants. Strengthens immune system and improves skin health.

18. **Bok Choy**
    Benefits: Contains selenium and vitamin K. Supports thyroid health and detoxification pathways.

19. **Turnip Greens**
    Benefits: High in calcium, vitamin A, and antioxidants. Supports bone and eye health.

20. **Ginger (root, used in small amounts)**
    Benefits: A powerful anti-inflammatory and digestive aid. Stimulates circulation and relieves nausea and muscle soreness.

Fruits for Juicing & Their Health Benefits

1. **Lemon**
    Benefits: Detoxifies the liver, alkalizes the body, boosts vitamin C, and supports digestion.

2. **Apple (especially green)**
   Benefits: Rich in fiber and antioxidants. Helps regulate blood sugar and supports gut health.

3. **Pineapple**
   Benefits: Contains bromelain, which aids digestion and reduces inflammation. High in vitamin C.

4. **Orange**
   Benefits: Loaded with vitamin C and potassium. Boosts immunity and supports skin and heart health.

5. **Blueberries**
   Benefits: Packed with antioxidants and phytonutrients. Supports brain health and reduces oxidative stress.

6. **Watermelon**
   Benefits: Extremely hydrating and contains citrulline, which supports blood flow and detoxification.

7. **Grapefruit**
   Benefits: Aids fat burning, supports liver function, and is high in vitamin C and antioxidants.

8. **Strawberries**
   Benefits: High in vitamin C and fiber. Supports skin health, reduces inflammation, and protects the heart.

9. **Kiwi**
   Benefits: Rich in vitamin C, E, and digestive enzymes. Supports immunity and gut health.

10. **Mango**
    Benefits: Full of vitamin A and digestive enzymes. Supports eye health, digestion, and skin glow.

11. **Papaya**
    Benefits: Contains papain, which aids digestion. Helps with inflammation and supports glowing skin.

12. **Pomegranate**
    Benefits: High in polyphenols and antioxidants. Supports heart health and fights inflammation.

13. **Cranberries (unsweetened)**
    Benefits: Helps prevent urinary tract infections, supports gut health, and is rich in antioxidants.

14. **Banana (best in smoothies)**
    Benefits: Rich in potassium and vitamin B6. Provides sustained energy and supports muscle recovery.

15. **Blackberries**
    Benefits: High in fiber and antioxidants. Supports brain health, detoxification, and cellular repair.

16. **Cherries**
    Benefits: Reduce inflammation and muscle soreness. Supports better sleep and joint health.

17. **Grapes (especially red or purple with seeds)**
    Benefits: Contain resveratrol, which supports heart and brain health and has anti-aging effects.

18. **Peaches**
    Benefits: High in vitamins A and C. Support skin health, digestion, and immune strength.

19. **Cantaloupe (melon)**
    Benefits: Very hydrating, high in beta-carotene. Supports immune function and skin repair.

20. **Dragon Fruit (Pitaya)**
    Benefits: Rich in vitamin C, fiber, and antioxidants. Supports gut health and boosts energy levels.

Fruits and Vegetables Juicing Ideas
Knowing which fruit and vegetables to put together to get great health benefits but also a great taste can be challenging for those new to juicing. Here are some combos to get you started.

1. Green Glow Juice

- Apple

- Cucumber

- Spinach

- Lemon

- Ginger
    Light, refreshing, and great for digestion and glowing skin.

2. Morning Sunshine Juice

- Carrot

- Orange

- Pineapple

- Turmeric (small piece or powder)
    Immunity-boosting and energizing with natural sweetness.

3. Berry Fresh Juice

- Strawberries

- Cucumber

- Celery

- Mint leaves
  Hydrating and antioxidant-rich with a hint of sweetness.

4. Tropical Greens Juice

- Pineapple

- Kale

- Green apple

- Lime
  Sweet, tangy, and packed with vitamin C and chlorophyll.

5. Summer Hydration Juice

- Watermelon

- Mint

- Cucumber

- Lime
  Very hydrating, anti-inflammatory, and great for hot days.

6. Apple Carrot Zinger

- Carrots

- Apples

- Ginger

- Lemon
  A classic combo that's sweet with a spicy kick—great for energy and digestion.

7. Purple Power Juice

- Red grapes

- Red cabbage

- Blueberries

- Lemon
  Antioxidant-rich and deliciously vibrant with a bold flavor.

8. Pear & Greens Refresh

- Pear

- Romaine lettuce

- Cucumber

- Parsley
  Mild, refreshing, and great for skin and hydration.

---

9. Strawberry Lemonade Greens

- Strawberries

- Lemon

- Spinach

- Apple
  Tastes like strawberry lemonade with a green boost.

---

10. Golden Glow Juice

- Pineapple

- Carrot

- Small piece of sweet potato

- Ginger
  Rich in beta-carotene and vitamin A, with a smooth and naturally sweet flavor.

Chapter 5: Juicing Tips and Precautions

- Use organic produce when possible to avoid pesticides.
- Drink juice immediately to preserve nutrients.
- Don't rely solely on juice; maintain a balanced diet.
- Listen to your body and adjust ingredients based on how you feel.

Why You Should Use Organic Produce for Juicing: Protecting Your Health from Pesticides

Juicing is a powerful way to deliver concentrated nutrition to the body. With each glass, you're extracting the vitamins, minerals, enzymes, and antioxidants from fruits and vegetables in their purest liquid form. But if you're not mindful about the quality of your produce, you may also be drinking something you don't want—**pesticides**. That's why choosing **organic produce whenever possible** is essential when juicing, not just for better flavor, but for better health.

The Problem with Pesticides

Conventional (non-organic) fruits and vegetables are often treated with synthetic pesticides and herbicides during farming. These chemicals are designed to kill pests, mold, or weeds—but they can also have negative effects on the human body. Over time, **pesticide exposure has been linked to hormonal disruption, nervous system damage, digestive problems, fertility issues**, and even an increased risk of certain cancers.

When you juice produce, you're consuming a **concentrated form** of whatever is on or inside that plant—including its chemicals. Unlike cooking, which can sometimes reduce pesticide residue, juicing keeps everything raw and uncooked. That means **whatever pesticides are on the skin or absorbed into the plant's flesh will end up in your juice.**

Why Organic Is Better

Organic produce is grown without synthetic pesticides, herbicides, or genetically modified organisms (GMOs). Farmers who grow organic crops use natural methods for pest control and soil health, such as compost, crop rotation, and beneficial insects. This results in **cleaner produce**—and cleaner juice.

When you choose organic, you're avoiding:

- Harmful pesticide residues

- Potential chemical build-up in your body

- Long-term exposure to toxins that can burden your liver and organs

Juicing is often done with the intention of detoxing and cleansing the body. Drinking pesticide-laden juice can do the opposite—it may actually add more toxins for your body to process.

Best Produce to Buy Organic

While going fully organic is ideal, it's not always affordable or possible for everyone. In that case, focus on organic versions of the **"Dirty Dozen"**—a list published by the Environmental Working Group (EWG) that identifies produce with the highest pesticide levels. These typically include:

- Strawberries

- Spinach

- Apples

- Grapes

- Celery

- Peaches

- Pears

- Cherries

- Tomatoes

- Bell peppers

- Kale

- Nectarines

Fruits and vegetables with **thin skins** or **that are eaten whole** are more likely to retain pesticide residue. On the other hand, produce like bananas, avocados, and pineapples (with thick peels) tend to have lower pesticide levels and are safer to buy conventionally.

Support for Long-Term Wellness

Using organic produce for juicing supports more than just your own body. It helps protect **farmworkers from chemical exposure**, promotes **environmentally friendly farming practices**, and reduces pollution in soil and water systems. By investing in organic products when you can, you're making a long-term investment in your health, the environment, and a more sustainable food system.

Great! Here's a simple, printable-style guide you can use or turn into a page for your wellness book, juicing guide, or fridge magnet:

Clean 15 vs. Dirty Dozen: Smart Organic Choices for Juicing

When juicing, **organic is best**—but if you're on a budget, this guide helps you decide **where to spend wisely** to avoid the most pesticides.

The Dirty Dozen

(*Buy these organic when possible — they have the highest pesticide residues*)

1. **Strawberries**

2. **Spinach**

3. **Apples**

4. **Grapes**

5. **Celery**

6. **Peaches**

7. **Pears**

8. **Cherries**

9. **Tomatoes**

10. **Bell Peppers & Hot Peppers**

11. **Kale, Collard & Mustard Greens**

12. **Nectarines**

The Clean 15

(Lower in pesticide residues — okay to buy non-organic if needed)

1. **Avocados**

2. **Sweet Corn**

3. **Pineapple**

4. **Onions**

5. **Papaya**

6. **Garlic**

7. **Cabbage**

8. **Kiwi**

9. **Honeydew Melon**

10. **Carrots**

11. **Watermelon**

12. **Mangoes**

13. **Sweet Potatoes**

14. **Bananas**

15. **Mushrooms**

💡 **Tips for Juicing on a Budget:**

- Prioritize organic for items on the **Dirty Dozen**.

- Peel thick-skinned conventional produce to reduce residue.

- Wash all fruits and veggies thoroughly—even organic ones.

- Shop local farmers' markets for affordable organic options.

- Buy in-season and freeze extra organic produce for juicing later.

Why You Should Drink Fresh Juice Immediately: Preserving Nutrients for Maximum Health Benefits

Juicing is one of the most effective ways to nourish your body with concentrated vitamins, minerals, and antioxidants straight from fruits and vegetables. Each glass of fresh juice can deliver a powerful dose of natural energy, immune support, and detoxifying compounds. But to truly gain the full benefits of juicing, **timing matters.** Drinking your juice immediately after preparation is essential to preserving its nutritional value and maximizing its health effects.

Nutrients Begin to Break Down Quickly

Freshly made juice is alive with enzymes, antioxidants, and vitamins that start to degrade **within minutes** of exposure to air, light, and heat. This process is called **oxidation**, and it begins as soon as fruits and vegetables are cut or pressed. Just like an apple turns brown after it's sliced, nutrients in juice begin to break down when they come in contact with oxygen. The longer juice sits, the more nutritional value it loses.

For example:

- **Vitamin C**—a powerful antioxidant—can degrade by up to 50% within the first hour if juice is left unrefrigerated.

- **Enzymes**, which help with digestion and cellular repair, are sensitive to light and heat and lose effectiveness quickly.

- **Polyphenols** and other plant compounds may also diminish, reducing the anti-inflammatory and detoxifying effects of the juice.

Fresh Juice = Fresh Energy

Juice is often consumed to boost energy, improve focus, or support a healthy cleanse. Drinking your juice right away ensures that your body receives the **maximum amount of bioavailable nutrients**, which can be absorbed easily and used quickly. Fresh juice can help regulate blood sugar, hydrate your cells, and provide a natural energy lift—benefits that are strongest when the juice is consumed within minutes of being made.

Delayed Drinking = Diminished Benefits

The longer juice sits, the more it:

- **Loses flavor and color**

- Becomes **less effective as a detox or healing tool**

- May **spoil or ferment**, especially if not stored properly

- Can **develop bacteria** if left unrefrigerated

While it's possible to store juice in the fridge for a short time (especially if cold-pressed and properly sealed), nothing compares to the **freshness and potency** of juice consumed right after it's made.

How to Preserve Juice If You Must Store It

If you absolutely need to store juice for later, you can slow nutrient loss by:

- Using **a masticating (cold press) juicer**, which creates less heat and oxidation

- Storing juice in **an airtight glass container**

- **Filling the container to the top** to minimize air exposure

- Keeping it **refrigerated immediately**

- Adding a bit of **lemon juice** as a natural preservative

Even with these steps, juice is best consumed **within 24–48 hours**, and ideally within 4–6 hours for optimal nutrient retention.

Fresh juice can last **up to 3 months in the freezer** if stored properly, but for best taste and nutrition, it's ideal to consume it within **30 to 60 days**.

Tips for Freezing Fresh Juice:

- **Use airtight containers**: Glass jars (leave 1–2 inches of space for expansion) or BPA-free freezer-safe containers work best.

- **Portion it**: Freeze in small batches (like ice cube trays or 8–12 oz jars) for easy use.

- **Label it**: Include the date and ingredients.

- **Thaw in the fridge overnight**: Avoid microwaving to preserve nutrients.

🚫 What to Avoid:

- Don't refreeze thawed juice.

- Don't fill containers to the top—juice expands when frozen and can crack jars.

Nutrient Note:

While freezing slows nutrient loss, **some vitamin C and enzymes may degrade slightly** over time. However, frozen juice is still far better than store-bought varieties with preservatives.

Certainly! Here's an essay explaining why **natural juice should not be your only source of nutrition**, and why a **balanced diet is essential** for true, long-term health:

A Balanced Diet Matters for Lasting Health

Natural juice made from fresh fruits and vegetables is a powerful addition to any healthy lifestyle. It floods the body with vitamins, minerals, antioxidants, and enzymes that support detoxification, boost energy, and nourish cells. However, while juicing offers many benefits, it should never be relied on as your sole source of nutrition. To experience true, lasting health, your body needs a **diverse, balanced diet** that includes a variety of whole foods beyond what juice alone can provide.

The Limits of Juice

Juicing removes most of the fiber from fruits and vegetables—one of the key components that helps regulate digestion, blood sugar, and satiety. Fiber is essential for:

- Supporting gut health

- Reducing cholesterol

- Stabilizing blood sugar levels

- Keeping you full and satisfied

Without fiber, juice is digested very quickly. This can lead to **spikes and crashes in blood sugar**, especially if the juice is high in fruit and low in greens or vegetables. Over time, consuming only juice without the fiber and structure of whole foods can lead to nutrient imbalances and cravings.

Missing Key Nutrients

While juice is rich in **vitamins, minerals, and antioxidants**, it often lacks:

- **Protein**, which is essential for muscle repair, immune function, and hormone production

- **Healthy fats**, which support brain function, cell health, and absorption of fat-soluble vitamins (A, D, E, and K)

- **Complex carbohydrates**, which provide long-lasting energy and support metabolic health

These nutrients can't be delivered in meaningful amounts through juice alone. That's why a well-rounded diet including **lean proteins, whole grains, healthy fats, legumes, and fiber-rich vegetables** is essential.

The Risk of Over-Reliance

Relying solely on juice can:

- Lead to **muscle loss** if protein intake is too low

- Cause **fatigue or mood swings** due to unstable blood sugar

- Slow metabolism over time if calorie intake is too low

- Cause nutritional deficiencies, especially in iron, calcium, and omega-3 fatty acids

- Be unsustainable, leading to **yo-yo dieting** or poor eating habits once juice-only plans end

While short-term juice cleanses may give your body a temporary reset, they should not replace consistent, balanced eating habits.

The Power of a Balanced Approach

Juicing is best used as a **supplement** to a healthy diet—not a substitute. A balanced diet includes:

- **Whole vegetables and fruits** (raw, cooked, or blended for fiber)

- **Whole grains** like quinoa, brown rice, and oats

- **Nuts, seeds, and healthy oils** for fats

- **Protein sources** such as beans, eggs, poultry, tofu, or fish

- Plenty of **water** and other hydrating fluids

- Occasional juices to boost nutrients, detoxify, or energize

This approach helps maintain healthy digestion, strong immunity, muscle tone, energy balance, and mental focus.

Listen to Your Body: Adjusting Your Juice Ingredients for Personal Health and Balance

Juicing is a wonderful way to support your health with natural nutrients, enzymes, and hydration. It can energize the body, cleanse the system, and even help improve digestion, skin clarity, and immune strength. But just like any health practice, juicing isn't one-size-fits-all. Everyone's body is different—what feels good and healing to one person may cause discomfort for another. That's why one of the most important rules in juicing is simple: **listen to your body.** Pay attention to how you feel after drinking certain juice blends, and be willing to adjust your ingredients to meet your body's unique needs.

Your Body Sends Signals—Pay Attention

When you drink juice, your body responds quickly. You may feel energized, lighter, and refreshed. Or, you might feel bloated, lightheaded, or even tired. These reactions are **signals**—your body's way of communicating what's working and what's not.

For example:

- If you feel **jittery or anxious** after drinking a fruit-heavy juice, your blood sugar may be spiking. Try using fewer fruits and adding more greens or fiber-rich veggies.

- If you feel **bloated or uncomfortable**, your juice may be too cold, too acidic, or contain ingredients your gut doesn't like (like cabbage or kale in some people).

- If you feel **nourished and calm**, that may be a sign you've found a good balance of ingredients for your current needs.

No "Perfect" Recipe for Everyone

Health trends often promote "superfoods" or "perfect juice recipes," but the truth is, **what works for one person might not work for another.** Your age, activity level, health conditions, stress levels, and even the season of the year can influence what your body needs.

For example:

- A person with **low blood sugar** might feel better with juices that include healthy fats (like avocado in a smoothie or a splash of coconut milk).

- Someone dealing with **inflammation** might benefit more from turmeric, ginger, and leafy greens.

- If you're feeling **sluggish or cold**, warming ingredients like ginger, lemon, or a small amount of cayenne pepper can help stimulate circulation and energy.

Start Simple, Then Adjust

If you're new to juicing, start with **simple blends**—maybe just 2 or 3 ingredients. Monitor how you feel for an hour or two afterward. Do you feel energized? Calm? Craving more sugar? Once you understand your response, you can gradually experiment by:

- Adding or removing ingredients

- Changing the fruit-to-veggie ratio

- Including herbs or spices like mint, parsley, or turmeric

- Adjusting for taste, digestion, or energy needs

Keeping a small **juice journal** can be helpful—note what you drank, how it tasted, and how you felt afterward.

Health Isn't Just About Recipes—It's About Connection

The most powerful part of juicing is not just the nutrients—it's the opportunity to **reconnect with your body**. Tuning into how your body responds builds awareness and teaches you to trust your internal signals. This practice goes beyond juicing—it can improve how you eat, move, sleep, and live.

Great! Below is a **printable-style "Listen to Your Body" Juice Journal Page** and a simple **Juice Adjustment Guide** based on how you feel after drinking your juice. You can use these as part of a book, PDF handout, or personal wellness tool.

Juice Adjustment Guide: How to Fine-Tune Based on How You Feel

If You Feel...	What It Might Mean	Try This Adjustment
Bloated	Juice may be too cold, acidic, or fibrous	Use more cucumber or zucchini; avoid cabbage/kale for a while
Jittery or Lightheaded	Blood sugar spike from too much fruit	Add more greens and fiber-rich veggies; reduce sweet fruits
Still hungry after juicing	Lacking protein or fat	Pair with a boiled egg, smoothie, or handful of nuts
Craving sugar soon after	Fruit-heavy juice causing blood sugar crash	Include lemon, celery, greens, or cinnamon for balance
Sluggish or tired	Body may need iron, or juice wasn't nutrient-dense enough	Add spinach, beet, or spirulina; reduce starchy vegetables
Gassy or uncomfortable	Certain veggies don't agree with your gut	Eliminate one suspect at a time (e.g., broccoli, cabbage, beets)
Glowing skin and energy boost	Great combo for your body!	Note the ingredients and make it a regular part of your routine

Chapter 6: Benefits and Precautions of Juice Fasting

Key Points – Benefits and Precautions of Juice Fasting

- Juice fasting can help detoxify the body, reset digestion, and increase mental clarity.

- It provides a quick influx of vitamins and antioxidants but may lack protein and fiber.

- Short-term juice fasts can boost energy and reduce cravings, but long-term fasting may cause nutrient imbalances.

- Juice fasting is not suitable for everyone and should be approached with care, especially for those with medical conditions.

Juice Fasting: Benefits and Precautions for a Balanced Detox

Juice fasting, the practice of consuming only fruit and vegetable juices for a period of time, has grown in popularity among those seeking to detoxify their bodies, reset their digestion, and jumpstart a healthier lifestyle. While juice fasting offers many potential health benefits, it also comes with important considerations. It is not a one-size-fits-all approach and should be done with mindfulness, preparation, and respect for your body's individual needs.

Benefits of Juice Fasting

1. **Detoxification and Organ Support**
   Juice fasting allows the digestive system to take a break from heavy processing. By consuming only nutrient-dense juices, the body can redirect energy toward detoxification and cellular repair. Ingredients like beetroot,

lemon, ginger, and celery support liver and kidney function, helping the body flush out accumulated toxins more efficiently.

2. **Increased Nutrient Absorption**
   Juices are absorbed more rapidly than whole foods, delivering a quick burst of vitamins, minerals, and antioxidants directly to your bloodstream. This can be especially helpful for people who have poor nutrient absorption due to digestive issues. Green juices rich in chlorophyll also support blood oxygenation and cellular regeneration.

3. **Improved Mental Clarity and Energy**
   Many people report heightened focus, lighter moods, and greater energy levels during a juice fast. This may result from removing processed foods, added sugars, and caffeine from the diet, as well as the anti-inflammatory and alkalizing effects of fresh juice.

4. **Resetting Cravings and Taste Buds**
   Juice fasting can help reduce cravings for junk food, sugar, and stimulants. After just a few days, your palate may become more sensitive, making you appreciate the natural flavors of fruits, vegetables, and whole foods again. It also encourages mindfulness about what you put into your body.

Precautions and Potential Drawbacks

1. **Lack of Protein and Fiber**
   Juice fasting eliminates fiber, which is crucial for digestion, blood sugar regulation, and satiety. It also contains little to no protein or healthy fat, which are necessary for muscle repair, hormone production, and long-term energy. Extended fasting without these macronutrients can lead to fatigue, muscle loss, or weakened immunity.

2. **Blood Sugar Spikes**
   Juices made primarily from fruit can cause rapid increases in blood sugar,

especially if consumed without fiber or protein. This can result in energy crashes, mood swings, and even dizziness. To prevent this, it's best to use more vegetables than fruits and include ingredients like lemon, cucumber, and leafy greens.

3. **Temporary Side Effects**

    Headaches, fatigue, irritability, and digestive discomfort are common in the first 1–3 days of a juice fast. These are often signs of detoxification, caffeine withdrawal, or electrolyte imbalances. Staying hydrated and getting adequate rest can help minimize these effects.

4. **Not Suitable for Everyone**

    Juice fasting is not recommended for children, pregnant or breastfeeding women, people with diabetes, eating disorders, or chronic health conditions unless supervised by a healthcare provider. Even healthy individuals should limit juice fasts to short durations (1–3 days) unless under professional guidance.

Chapter 7 Start Juicing Today

Why You Should Start Juicing: A Simple Step Toward a Healthier You

In a world where fast food and processed snacks are more accessible than ever, people are growing more disconnected from real, nourishing foods. As a result, chronic fatigue, digestive issues, and preventable diseases are on the rise. But there's a simple, natural solution that can help restore your body, boost your energy, and enhance your well-being: **juicing**. Drinking fresh juice made from raw fruits and vegetables is not only delicious, it's one of the most effective ways to give your body the nutrients it truly craves. **If you care about your health, you should absolutely start juicing.**

Juicing Delivers Powerful Nutrition Fast

Juicing provides an **instant dose of vitamins, minerals, and antioxidants**—without the burden of heavy digestion. Because juice is liquid, your body can absorb nutrients quickly and efficiently. In just one glass, you can drink the equivalent of several servings of fruits and vegetables. This makes juicing perfect for busy people who may not have time to sit down to multiple healthy meals every day. Juicing doesn't just fill you up—it **fuels you**.

Juicing Helps Cleanse and Heal the Body

Our bodies are constantly bombarded by toxins from processed food, pollution, and stress. Juicing helps flush out these toxins by giving your organs, especially the **liver and kidneys**, a break from processing chemicals and waste. Ingredients like beets, dandelion root, lemon, and celery are known to support the body's natural detoxification processes. Regular juicing can lead to clearer skin, improved digestion, and even weight loss—all signs your body is healing from the inside out.

Feel the Difference in Energy and Focus

One of the biggest benefits people notice when they start juicing is a **burst of natural energy**. Unlike caffeine or sugar highs, juice gives you a clean, steady boost without the crash. Nutrient-rich juices feed your cells, oxygenate your blood, and support better brain function. If you often feel tired, foggy, or sluggish, juicing can help you feel more alert, focused, and alive.

Juicing Can Reset Cravings and Eating Habits

Many people struggle with unhealthy cravings for sugar, salty snacks, and junk food. Juicing helps retrain your palate and **reduce cravings naturally**. When your body gets the nutrients it needs, you feel satisfied on a cellular level—making it easier to say no to processed foods. Juicing can be the gateway to a healthier lifestyle by helping you crave more whole, real foods.

It's an Act of Self-Care and Mindfulness

Choosing to juice means you're choosing to put your health first. It's a small daily ritual that says, "My body is worth taking care of." In a world full of quick fixes and empty calories, juicing reconnects you with the power of **natural, living food**. It can become a grounding, mindful practice that helps you feel centered, present, and in control of your health.

Start Juicing, Start Thriving

Juicing isn't a fad—it's a **smart, simple, and powerful habit** that can change your health and your life. It gives your body the tools it needs to heal, energize, and thrive in a natural, sustainable way. Whether you want to boost your energy, improve digestion, clear your skin, or just feel better overall, juicing is a step in the right direction. So don't wait. **Grab your juicer, load up on vibrant produce, and give your body the gift of real nourishment.** You'll feel the difference—and your future self will thank you.

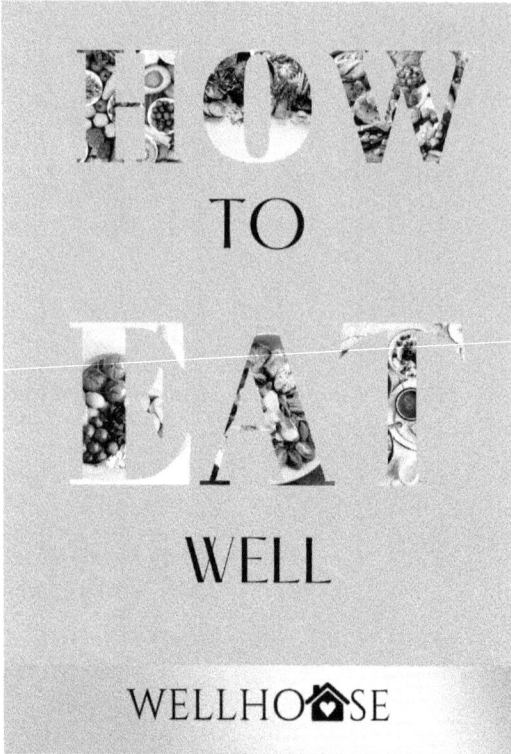

HOW TO EAT WELL

WELLHOUSE

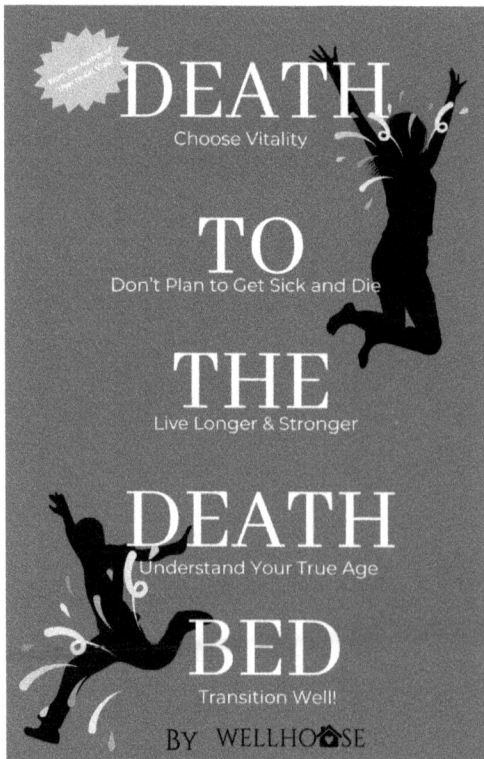

DEATH
Choose Vitality

TO
Don't Plan to Get Sick and Die

THE
Live Longer & Stronger

DEATH
Understand Your True Age

BED
Transition Well!

BY WELLHOUSE

www.ingramcontent.com/pod-product-compliance
Lightning Source LLC
Chambersburg PA
CBHW070031030426
42335CB00017B/2388